Navigating Your Transplant Journey

From Referral to Living Life Again

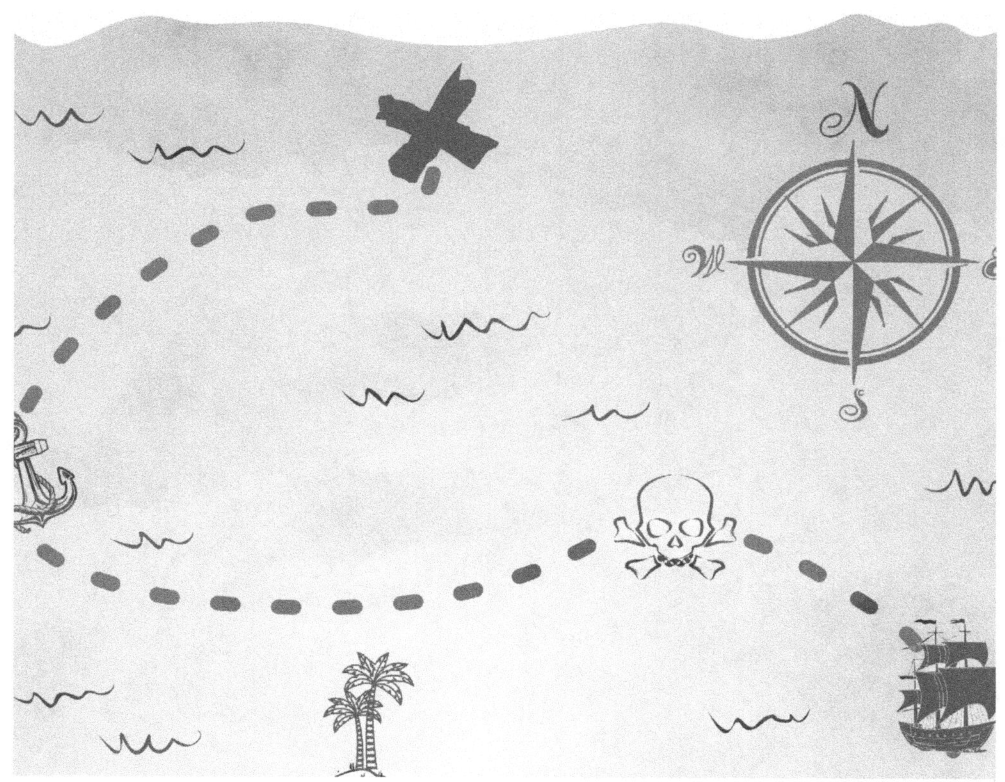

Beth Campbell Duke ~ TransplantRogues.com

Navigating Your Transplant Journey

Foreword: About Tony & Beth

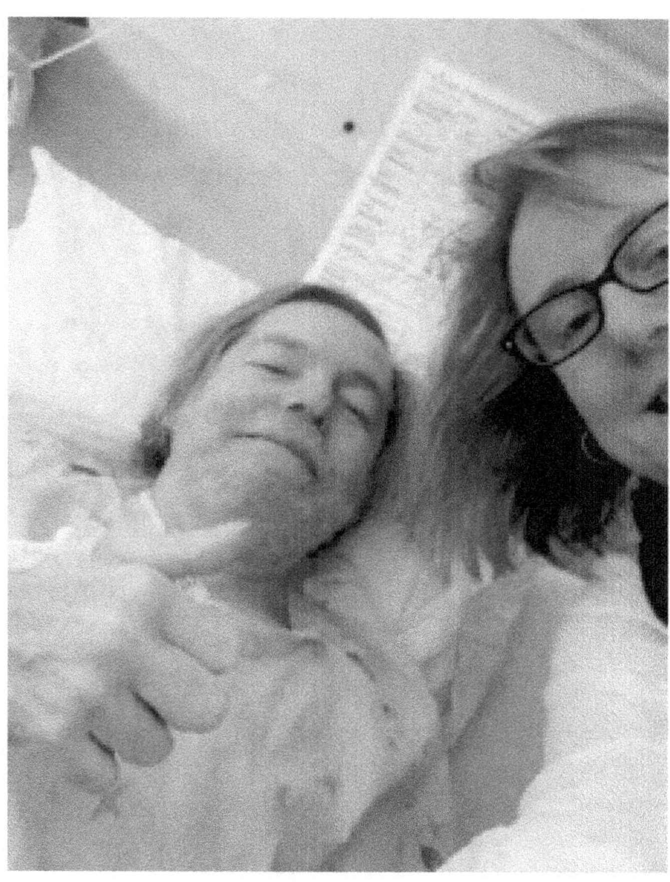

This is us in the Step-Down Unit after Tony's double-lung transplant at Vancouver General Hospital in Canada. This was May 2016.

When Tony's not being a Transplant Rogue, he works as an antique and personal property appraiser. Antiques are in his blood. He grew up in the trade, working as a French Polisher, an auctioneer as well as running shops. He's also been an 'expert' on the Canadian Antiques Roadshow and has kept his ID badge to prove it.

Beth is an ex-biotechie and high-school-teacher-dropout. She left teaching when they moved from Saskatchewan in 2008 - because the winters were too cold for Tony's lungs and they were seriously concerned for his health. Back then his diagnosis was 'asthma'. Since moving to British Columbia, Beth has been trying to find her own niche - first in helping Tony promote his antique services (until his health became too poor) and then using her teaching experience to help people in the area of careers. Now in the transplant community, she knows she's finally landed. This workbook combines both of Beth's backgrounds - science and education.

Getting to transplant and rebuilding your life afterwards is a long road. Think marathon. Like running a long race, there will be easier times and then times you hit the wall and wonder if you can go on. You can.

You've Got This!

Disclaimer

This workbook doesn't offer medical advice. Its purpose is to help you navigate your Transplant Journey. This is a journey that involves the transplant candidate/recipient as well as family, friends and caregivers - and of course, your medical team.

Each country and jurisdiction has different requirements, processes and support mechanisms in place. We designed this workbook based on our own experience with Tony's double lung transplant in British Columbia Canada. If you live elsewhere, you can use this book as a reference and to help you formulate pro-active questions for your own Transplant Journey.

As you make your way through this workbook, you'll see that each section has instructions for incorporating the information you receive from your health-care and transplant teams. This workbook- and the patient binder it helps you pull together - is designed to be a document that evolves as you move through the process. It wants you to write on it and rearrange the sections according to your needs.

NB*: It's* <u>*critical*</u> *that you direct any and all medical questions to your primary care and transplant team members. This is their expertise and their role. Your transplant team is there to answer questions – you are not bothering them if you ask about something you previously might have thought of as a minor question. There's a lot to learn, and one of those things is that what might seem minor can be major. And vice versa. After transplant, it's a whole new ballgame.*

Smooth sailing. May your wait be short.

Preface: How to Use This Book

The information in this workbook is broken down into phases of the transplant journey.

We hope that this book can become your go-to resource during your journey - and that the patient binder we help you create can keep you organized. It will contain contact information, medical information, legal documents and other things you collect along the way – all in one spot.

As you use this workbook and develop your patient and caregiver binder, you'll be connected to your support systems and have information and plans in place.

There are 3 different kinds of pull-out boxes in this workbook with important information about system navigation, creating your binder and getting connected to yourself and your networks!

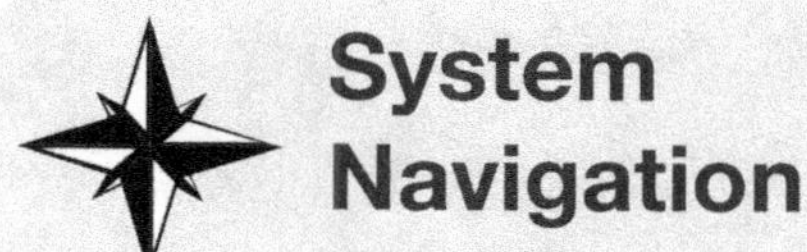
System Navigation

Includes information about our healthcare system as well as tips we learned along the way.

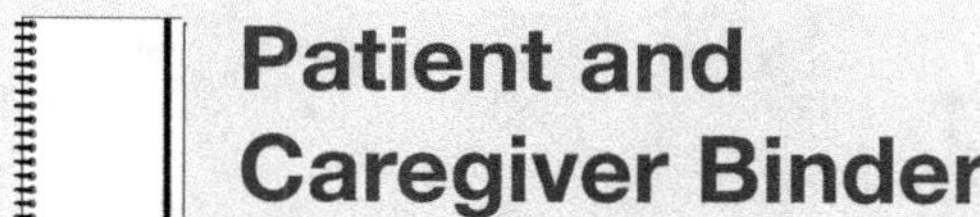
Patient and Caregiver Binder

Information that can help you get your healthcare information organized so communication with each other and your healthcare team members is easier.

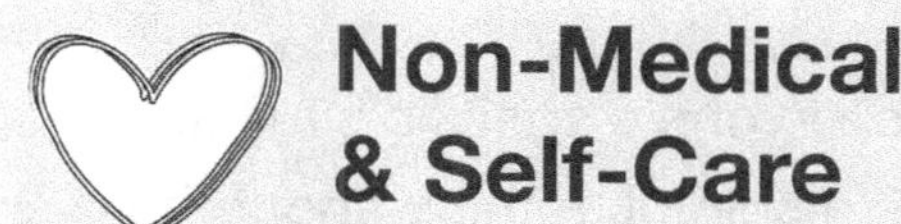
Non-Medical & Self-Care

This is the missing piece in the healthcare journey (at least for now). Nobody goes through a successful transplant journey without the support of others and picking up some wellness skills.

Map Out Your Journey

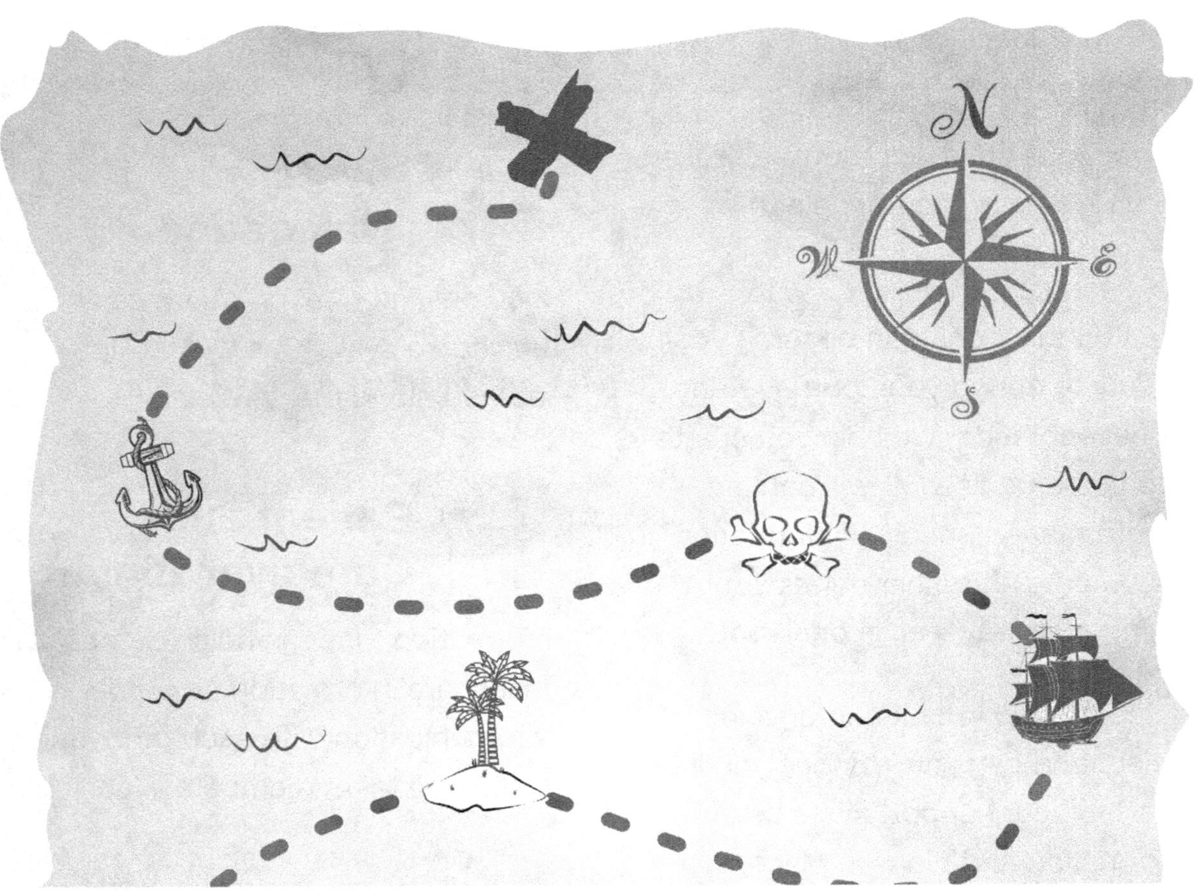

Because everyone's specific situation is different, it's helpful to think about the phases of the Transplant Journey with your situation in mind. This will help you map out the areas where you need to prepare, help you think about the kinds of questions you have, and start looking for the people who can/will help you.

Here's an example of the timeline from our own experience:

1. Tony spent a few years trying to **get a referral** for Transplant. He was told that he was too old at one point and only after we luckily had to move through a few GPs did we land with one seemed to take his requests seriously. ***What issues or questions do you have about getting a referral for transplant?***

2. It took 6 months from referral to our **first meeting with the Transplant Team**. We had no idea about planning anything at this stage (or following up with referrals), although we already had our legal documents in place. ***What questions would you have for your transplant team?***

3. We decided to proceed into **Pre-Transplant Assessment**. It took us 6 months to complete pre-transplant assessment, which is normal in our jurisdiction. In some countries you will be admitted to hospital and complete this step in 2-3 days. We also started thinking and talking about relocation for the transplant as we didn't live in or near Vancouver. ***What affairs need to be put in order during this time?***

4. **The Waiting List**. Aside from trying to sort out the logistics of making plans for an uncertain transplant date, and maintaining physical health to the best of your ability, the waiting list is a mental game. Social isolation may have been an issue before now, but it will ramp up here. ***How can you focus on maintaining an even keel while you're waiting?***

5. **Recovery Time in Hospital**. This is a scary and hopeful time. Trepidation and relief. The transplant recipient has a lot of support (and good drugs!). Beth was finally able to get some sleep at night. Because we had to relocate for 3 - 6 months, Beth had to find accommodation and she 'popped' home to get things sorted for the house-sitter. There will also be significant education for the patient and family to prepare for discharge. ***What will the caregiver need to get sorted during this time?***

6. **The First 3 Months**. When you're discharged, you are monitored very closely by your transplant team. We attended Transplant Clinic twice a week and a rehab program 3 times per week for 8 weeks. Not all organ transplants require the same followup care, so when you first meet with the transplant team be sure to ask: ***What***

will the first 3-6 months after transplant look like?

7. **The First Year: Rehab and Initial Recovery**. Transplant is a major medical intervention and a life-long chronic disease. You don't just 'bounce back'. Transplant requires continuous monitoring of vital signs to detect incidents of rejection and infection. The medications have side effects. There are medications for the side effects of your other medications. It's important to be on top of your own health. The realities of survival statistics will hit you as you will encounter bumps in the road, and some of your cohorts ~~may~~ will die. *How does your transplant clinic support patients and families? Is there support, or are you on your own?*

8. **The Second Year & Beyond: Defining Your New Normal**. Once we'd decided that we had to pack up and move, we made the decision to move not just 'into town', but to move to a bigger centre where we could better access medical programs, walk to stores and services and find work more easily. It took a toll selling the house and finding ourselves renting, but the move was necessary. We had a lot of issues to grapple with - and had to sort out our priorities. We figured it out and you will figure it out too! There will be good days and bad, but (fingers crossed) nothing like the issues that landed you on your transplant journey. You've got this. *What do you want your post-transplant life to look like?*

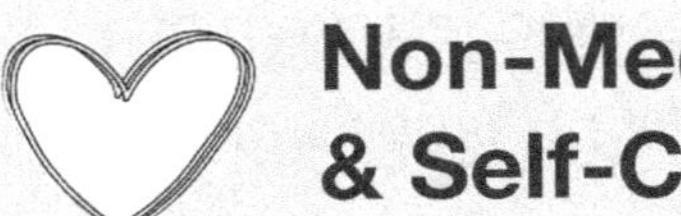

Non-Medical & Self-Care

You may have noticed a theme developing here about the absolute need for support. Social isolation was at the root of our significant depression issues post-transplant.

We now offer a series of workshops for patients and family caregivers that focus on system navigation and wellness. We use a fabulous tool I wish I'd known about **before** Tony's transplant that can help you *literally* map out your current medical and caregiving situation.

It's worth your time to sit down with a refreshing beverage and draw a CareMap: AtlasCareMap.org

Get connected with others in the transplant community online. Find us on Facebook: Facebook.com/TransplantRogues.

2

Getting the Referral

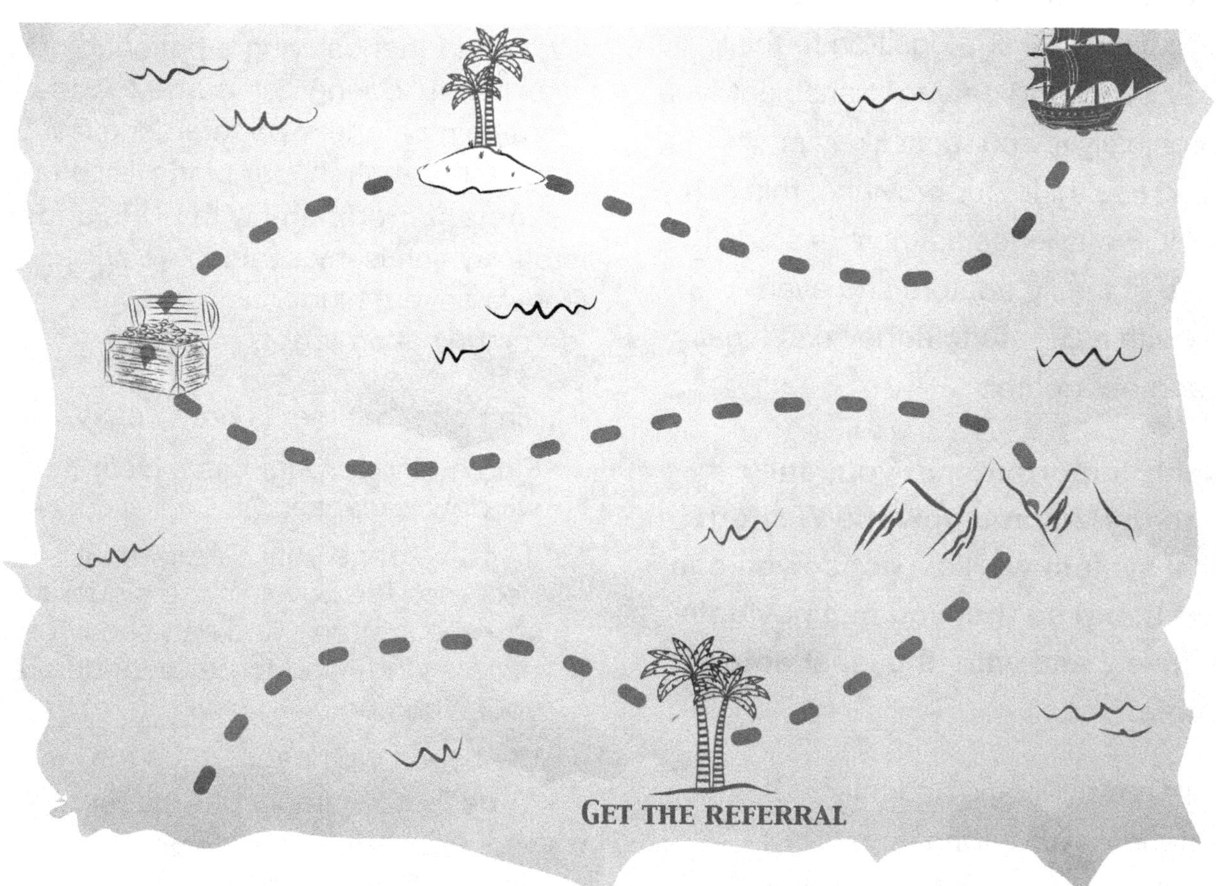

People's experiences of being referred for transplant vary.

In our case, Tony had inquired about transplant about 5 years before he was referred and he was told that he would never qualify for a transplant – yet when he was eventually referred he went through the Pre-Transplant Assessment stage with flying colours.

This was partly because things changed rapidly in the few years before Tony's transplant and because we landed with a new physician who seemed more knowledgable about the transplant process than the other GPs in the clinic.

From our experience, it's critical that you have a doctor with whom you can establish a good working relationship because if you are in a position to think you may be a candidate for transplant, you are chronically ill and most likely in declining health. In our province, this can be a HUGE challenge as there is a shortage of family doctors and even people with a GP are told they can't just go to another doctor.

It's highly important that you really begin to understand how the Western medical system works – not so you can change it, but so that you can navigate it effectively and with the least amount of trouble.

Be prepared for illogic and a lack of understanding about the impacts of chronic illness. Remember too, that doctors are busy and overworked. They need you to be prepared for appointments and be clear about why you're there.

Never confuse being tired of handling the nonsense of the system with an inability to handle it.

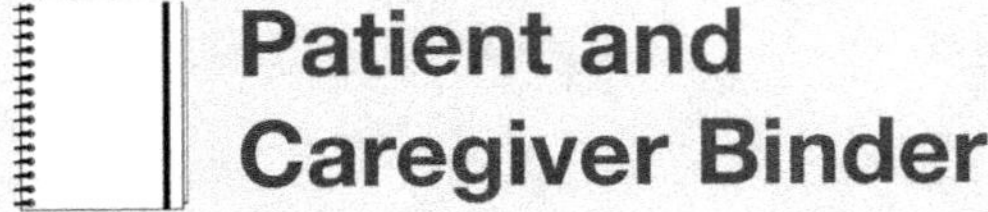

Patient and Caregiver Binder

Managing a critical and/or chronic illness requires patients and families to move up a steep learning curve. FAST. With no training.

We found that carrying a patient binder was helpful during our journey. Aside from being a one-stop reference for Tony's information, our binder also gave us **instant credibility** with EMTs and ER staff - which is invaluable. We still use Tony's patient binder as a communication tool.

Pulling one together is pretty easy:

1. Find a binder. Ours has a clear front window because...
2. If you've done your CareMap, it becomes the cover of the binder so you see it often - and can show it to people who need to better understand your situation.
3. We began with pages/tabs for:
   • A patient summary one-pager,
   • Contact info for members of your medical team and personal contacts,
   • Medications list, and
   • Clinic notes

We are often the **only ones** who carry our story and medical information among healthcare providers.

Help Your Doctor Refer You To Transplant

Many people tell stories of showing up at the doctor's or the Emergency Room, being seen by a doctor and immediately getting refered to the Transplant Team. If you would benefit from a transplant, that's the way you want it to happen.

But that's not always the case. Consider this: Transplantation is still in its relatively early years. It's growing by leaps and bounds, and not all doctors have had experience in identifying and referring potential candidates – in no small part because the definition of who is an acceptable candidate continues to expand.

The trick is that you have to either:

1. **Be seen by a doctor who is familiar with transplant criteria and the referral process, or**

2. **You need to help your doctor understand the transplant criteria and the referral process.**

Your GP plays a key role in your healthcare, and when if it comes to you needing a specialist, your GP is the 'gatekeeper'. If his or her practice is like the one we go to, he or she is seriously overworked. Our GP's office is only open for appointments Monday – Friday, but it is often staffed 7 days a week keeping up with the increasing expectations of a system that demands instant results.

Our GP still makes house-calls and he takes on chronically ill and elderly patients. The office staff call on Sundays to confirm Monday appointments. Or on Thanksgiving Monday to confirm a Tuesday appointment. Our GP has personally called in the evenings with blood test results from earlier in the day. It's not unheard of for him to call on a Sunday evening as he's preparing for the week – just to clarify issues or a test result. These people are busy, and they're going the extra mile for their patients.

Your doctor cannot be expected to know every medical detail on the planet Earth, and sometimes the staff will drop the ball. This is not personal. They are busy human beings.

If you are in the same position as Tony was 5 years ago, here's the bit we didn't know then:

• Our provincial transplant authority has published information on transplant criteria and the referral process online, and yours probably does, too! If you're going to be starting a Transplant Journey of your own, **now's the time to get very familiar with your transplant authority's website**. Look in the area for Health Professionals. As the patient or caregiver, you are now an unofficial Health Professional!

Consider Yourself Deputized

In our case, there are still no published guidelines for the referral of a patient for lung or liver transplant, but the guidelines for the other transplant organs are listed – and they all share the same broad criteria. (Find them here: BC Transplant Clinical Guidelines For Transplantation: http://www.transplant.bc.ca/health-professionals/clinical-guidelines).

Keep in mind that different transplant clinics can have very different selection and rejection criteria. As well, things change rapidly so a 'no' isn't always a 'no'. Sometimes getting listed for transplant requires tenacity. **It can be very difficult to know which bits are a hard 'no' and which bits are a flexible 'no'.** This is another reason to get connected to support within the transplant community.

Note also that two of these six criteria pertain to your social support network and willingness to comply. The social and mental health related aspects of getting listed for transplant are the ones we hear about in the patients and families community most frequently when people run into trouble getting listed. **There are many compelling reasons to get connected to support within the transplant community**.

Here are the broad criteria for transplant:

• **Progressive, irreversible disease**: you're sick and getting sicker and a transplant is the only option.

• **You have no active malignancy or infection**. Once transplanted, you will be on anti-rejection drugs for life. These are immuno-suppressants. If you have an active cancer, you aren't a candidate for transplant because you need your immune system at its top form to take care of the cancer. Having said that, this doesn't always disqualify you. Remember: Things are developing rapidly in the worlds of cancer and transplant.

• **There is an absence of systemic disease which would severely limit rehabilitation**: Transplant is major surgery and requires you to be otherwise healthy to cope with the surgery and physiotherapy during recovery.

• **Your life expectancy is reasonably greater than 5 years with a successful transplant**: This means that if you're older and otherwise healthy, you might not be too old! I had a woman stop by my donor registration booth recently whose sister-in-law had a liver transplant at 75. Buddy who was in the bed next to Tony on the lung transplant ward was 70.

• **You have effective family or social support systems**: There is a significant recovery period during which time the transplant patient requires a caregiver to make sure they understand what's required of them, take their meds at the right time and show up to appointments and rehab. Seriously, the high levels of anti-rejection meds and pain killers give recipients what our 'posse' calls CRS syndrome: Can't Remember $h!t Syndrome. One of Tony's comrades handed his wife a banana when she asked for the car keys. If you have to travel from your home to the city where the transplant is taking place it means relocating for a period of time. This means there can be significant financial barriers to getting listed that you will have to - and can - plan for.

Don't let all this throw you – when you have a chronic illness you're probably already used to seeing doctors and taking multiple medications. You may even have a good social support system. If not, you'll have a good start in doing a CareMap, and identifying strategies to get connected and find/ask for support.

There will be changes post-transplant – and you're most likely already establishing the habits you'll need to get through the process and life with a transplant.

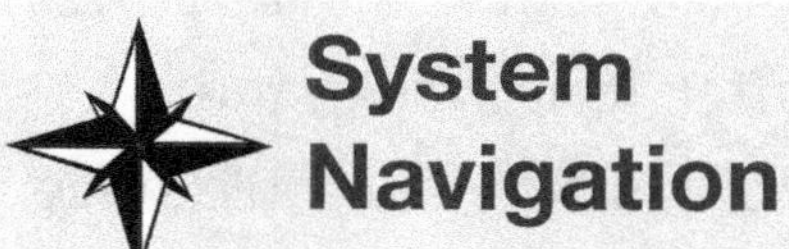

System Navigation

Determine a time period after which you will follow up when you get a referral to a specialist.

• Call the specialist's office to say 'hello' and double-check that they have received the referral. Add the contact info to your 'Members: My Transplant Team' sheet.

There are 2 reasons for this: these are new team members for you, and sometimes the referral gets forgotten or lost. You don't need the delay.

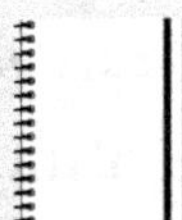

Patient & Caregiver Binder

• Using a formal system like the 'Clinic Notes' sheet included at the end of this workbook would have helped us organize our thoughts and questions more effectively and relieved some stress. Either one of us can add questions/concerns to be addressed at the next clinic or doctor's appointment and either of us can write in the answer and know what things need to be done.

• The 'Medication List' sheet included at the end of this workbook is in a format we adopted after Tony was in the hospital. Using this sooner would have helped us at doctor's appointments and when and ambulance had to be called, and it would have prevented a medication dosage error happening when he was admitted for transplant. The format of the medication list here is the one we ~~were provided with~~ stole when Tony was discharged.

Non-Medical & Self-Care

Special Note To Caregivers: This journey is a marathon. What you can carry for a short time is not at all sustainable for the long-haul that is transplant.

I wish I had realized the amount of ongoing caregiving that transplant requires. Tony's health declined over a period of time, so it was difficult to recognize and acknowledge my caregiving role. It meant switching my self-perception from partner to caregiver. For me it meant losing my partner and picking up his responsibilities in our day-to-day lives.

There currently is not a lot of societal recognition and support for caregivers, especially over the long-term. **You need support**.

Please create your own CareMap and patient binder. Ask for support from your family, friends, doctors and community groups. If you live in BC, AB, ON or NS find your Family Caregiver Association. It's **critically** important that you get connected to a support network. If you can't find or attend one locally, then find one online - whether it's through TransplantRogues.com or another

3

Meeting Your Transplant Team

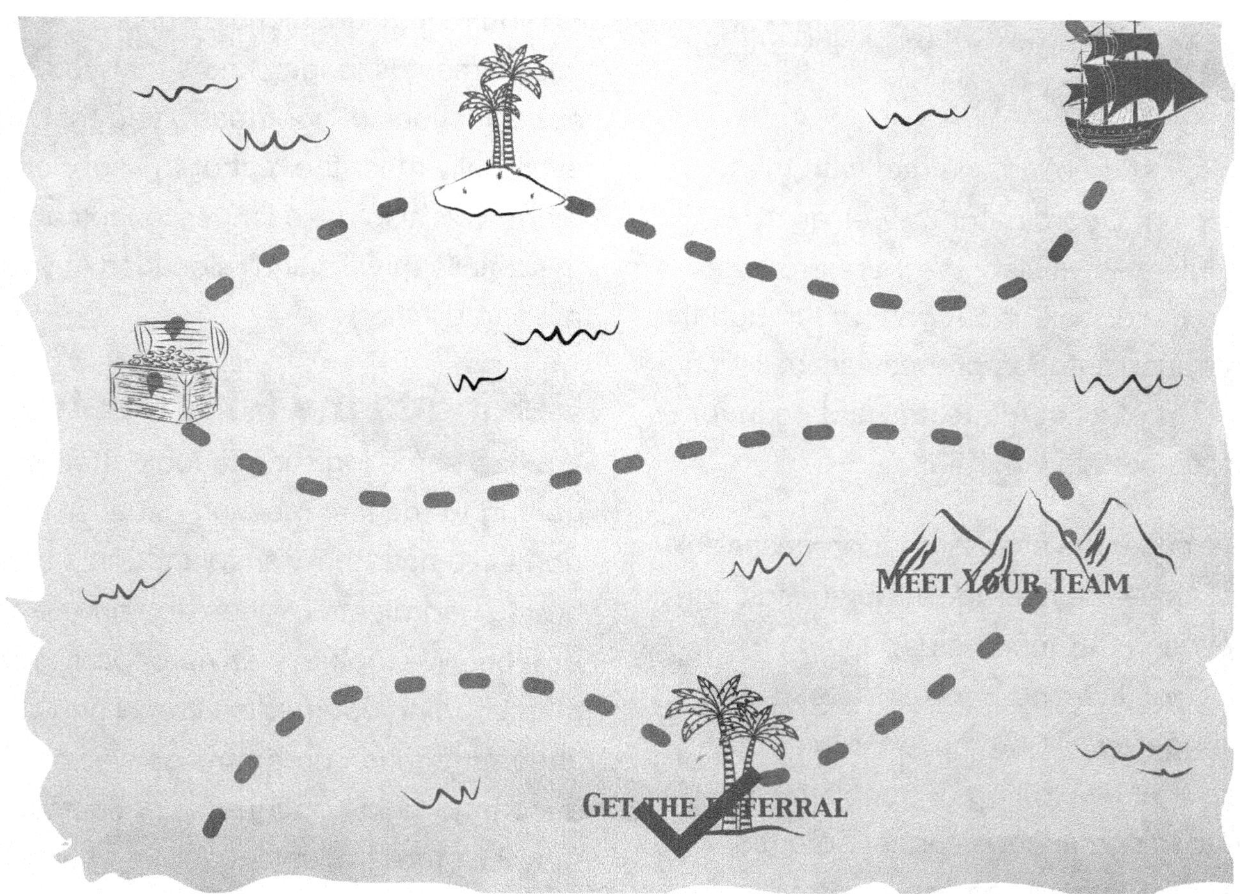

Aside from our GP, the Transplant Team were the first people in our journey to 'get us'. We were welcomed to the office and Tony was immediately offered an oxygen concentrator. That set the tone for us – as it had been a long time in even getting this meeting!

If you haven't felt this up until now: You've got people!

Our initial meeting was overwhelming.

There was a lot of nodding on our part and then we had questions after we got back to the hotel. Our main focus was in getting to the appointment and somehow making a good impression! We didn't want to be rejected and Tony's chronic illnesses made him especially sensitive to doctors who didn't want to take on his case. I can't tell you how relieved we were to land in the transplant clinic.

At this first meeting, we met with the Transplant Coordinator as well as a Transplant Physician. We were provided with a handbook about getting through the lung transplantation process as well as a checklist of all of the tests we'd be in for over the next few months.

In our case, the assessment process took 6 months – the average in our jurisdiction is between 3-6 months depending on where you live and what extra tests might get triggered as you move through the process. We've heard of people taking longer. In some jurisdictions, potential transplant candidates are admitted to the hospital and testing takes 3-4 days.

Now is the time to come prepared with any questions you may have. (Hopefully you have a number already written down from Chapter 1 and your CareMap.) At the end of the Pre-Assessment process we met with the larger transplant team:

• If you're in a jurisdiction that has the 3-4 day assessment period, you'll be moving through the next few stages quickly and you'll have a team to answer questions in short order. Have them ready!

• If you're in a jurisdiction where assessment is longer, know that you can ask questions of your team, and that you'll eventually meet the rest of the support team. You also have longer to look after the details of wills and relocation (if you have to do that).

Getting to the First Meeting

We had some logistics to look after in getting to the first meeting because we don't live near the Transplant Clinic and we had to coordinate oxygen equipment delivery. We took this as an opportunity to start scoping out medical travel and accommodation programs as well as accommodation options for patients and families. Your transplant authority and the hospital will likely have information for out-of-town patients and families. If you can't find them, call your transplant authority and hospital and ask for help finding this information! (Write the phone numbers onto your 'My Transplant Team' sheet. You'll need them again!)

Brainstorm the questions you want to ask during this first meeting if you haven't already done it, and write them down on a 'Clinic Notes' sheet. Here are some questions we wish we'd asked:

• How long does Pre-Transplant Assessment take?

• What kinds of tests are required? Are these done all at once or in phases? Is there a handout or list somewhere?

• How long is the hospitalization and follow-up? What is involved in the follow-up care?

• Do we need to relocate? For which parts? How do people usually find housing on short notice? How do they afford it?

• When we are listed for transplant, who are the members of the team?

• What should we be concentrating on during this time?

• What can we do to start getting ready for the next stage?

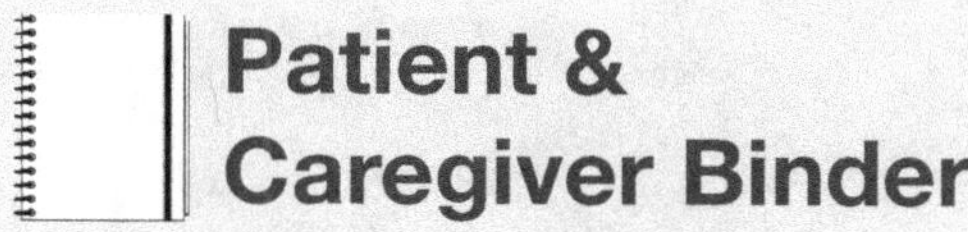

Take your binder with you to the first meeting. You'll get a lot of information!

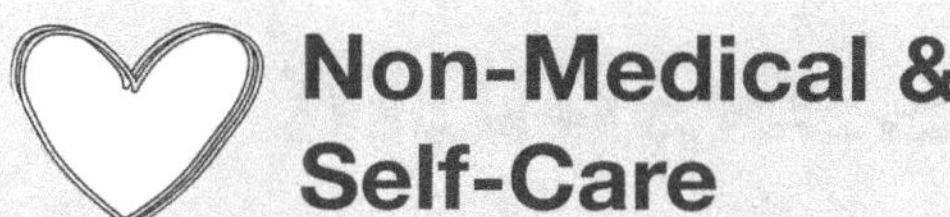

Get connected to us on Facebook if you're there. Let us know how it went!

Facebook.com/TransplantRogues

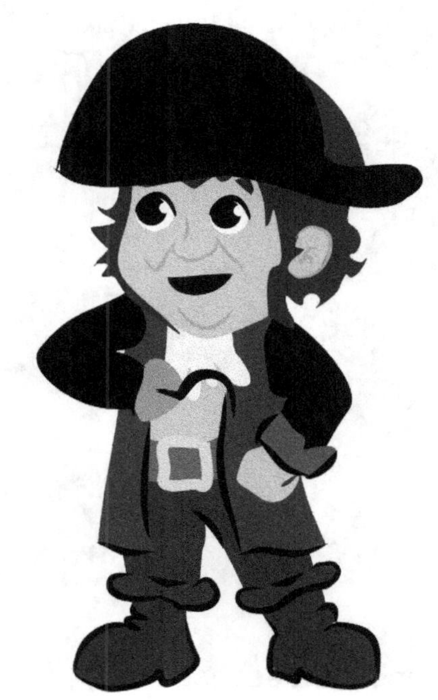

4

Pre-Transplant Assessment

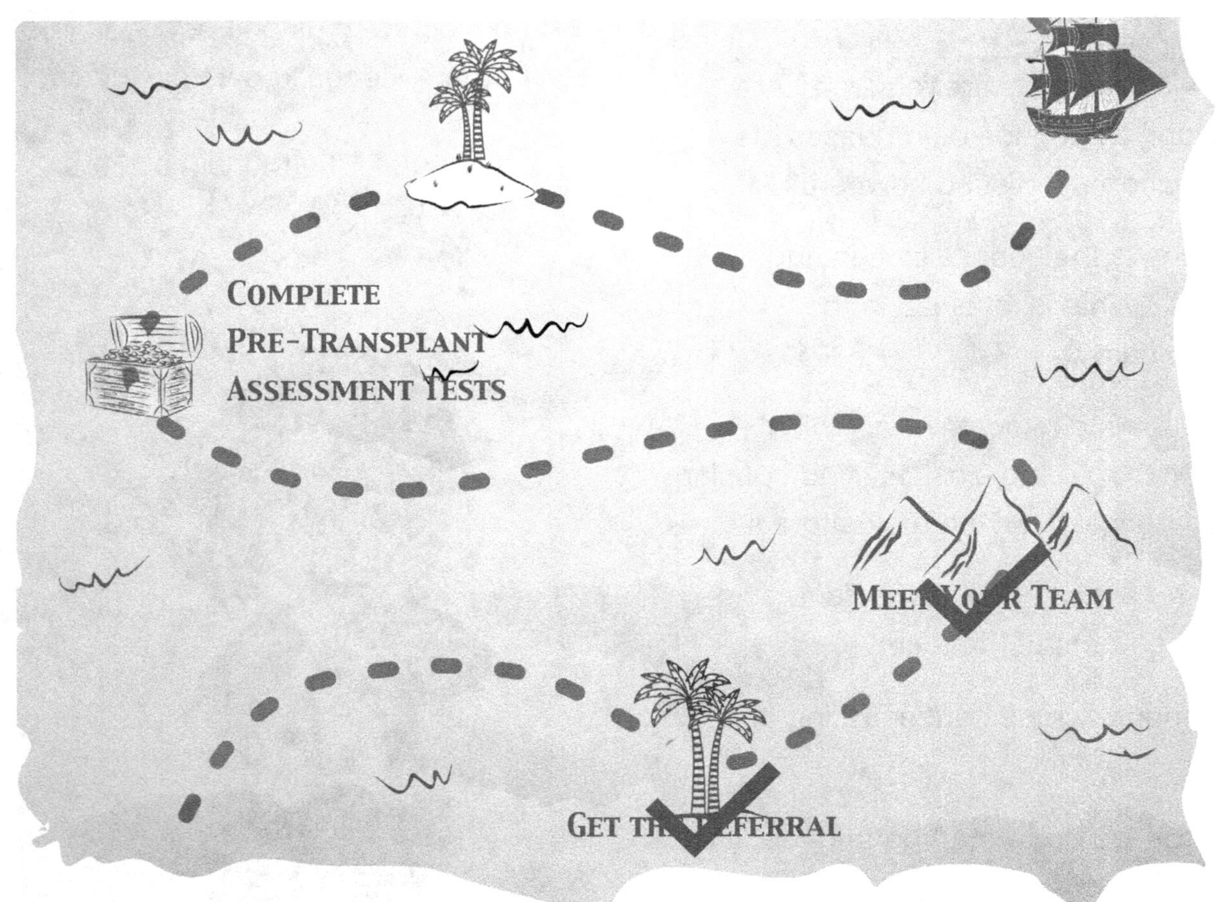

In pre-transplant assessment, you complete a battery of medical tests and sort out how to meet the non-medical criteria (i.e. finances and social supports/caregiver).

In our jurisdiction, tests are ordered in a hierarchical manner. We did the 'easy' ones first (blood tests, x-rays, CT scans) and when the results were in another 'phase' was ordered.

Tony had some extra tests ordered along the way. This is normal. The team isn't trying to eliminate you as a candidate so much as they absolutely need to get an accurate medical picture of what they're dealing with.

With all of these appointments to get to, there is a lot of running around and rebooking of appointments. With our local hospital there is no centralized booking system, so we had critical tests booked simultaneously and of course each lab believes they're the most important and you should 'just rebook' the other. There are sometimes wait-times that seem excessive and we often felt that the system just didn't understand the importance of getting these things done in a more efficient manner.

This is normal – so don't let it get you down. Find the coffee shop and get yourself a customer loyalty card right at the beginning.

Remember: A hospital is like a small village. Not everyone there has a medical background and even those who do don't always know about transplants - especially if you're going through assessment at a hospital that isn't your transplant hospital. You could well be the expert when it comes to the pre-transplant assessment process.

Pre-transplant assessment culminates with a meeting of the transplant team to determine whether they consider you a suitable candidate and if so, you decide whether you are willing to proceed.

At our final pre-transplant assessment meeting, we were also required to sign a number of consent and access to information forms and we had to provide a copy of Tony's Health Care Directive.

We had these already in place, and I had them with me as I had already used Tony's Power of Attorney documents because he was too ill to 'pop out' to sign things like car insurance, etc.

These last 'loose ends' have come as a surprise to some Rogues we've talked to who were feeling the weight of the process and thought they were done trying to check all the boxes for pre-transplant assessment.

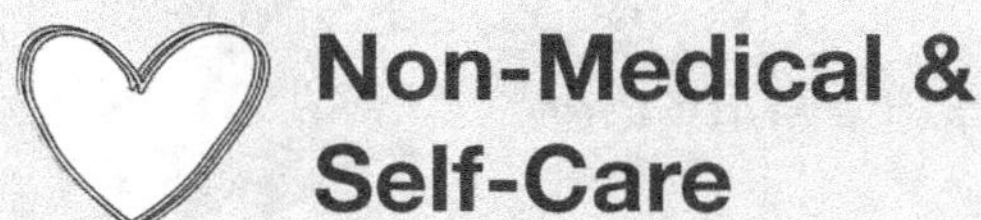

Non-Medical & Self-Care

This is a marathon, not a sprint. Find a support group and/or counsellor. ASAP.

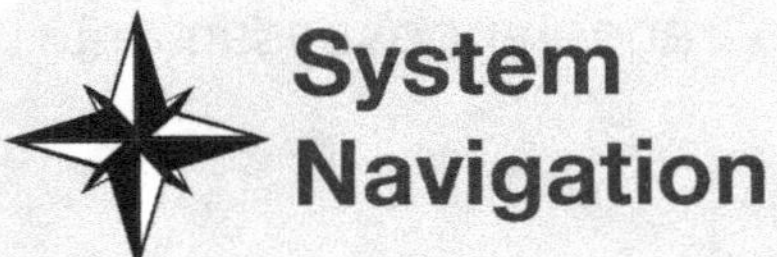

System Navigation

In Canada, Healthcare is a provincial responsibility. Mostly.

In our province, there are regional districts and our local hospital was no run by the health district, but by the Catholic Church.

Once we started to realize how many authorities were involved and got to be familiar with the staff at the front-lines it became easier to understand about the wait-times for testing and start to better explain to people at the hospital what the process was.

As we got to know people, they were often willing to look over our stack of orders and explain things.

Never forget that while your Transplant Team is doing fabulous work, they're probably like ours – a well-kept secret to others who have a hand in the process but don't realize it.

You're learning the ropes, but you're also an information-provider.

Remember: You've been deputized.

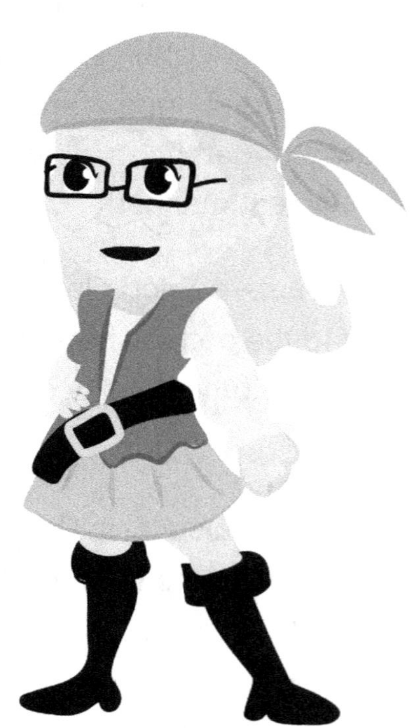

5

The Waiting List

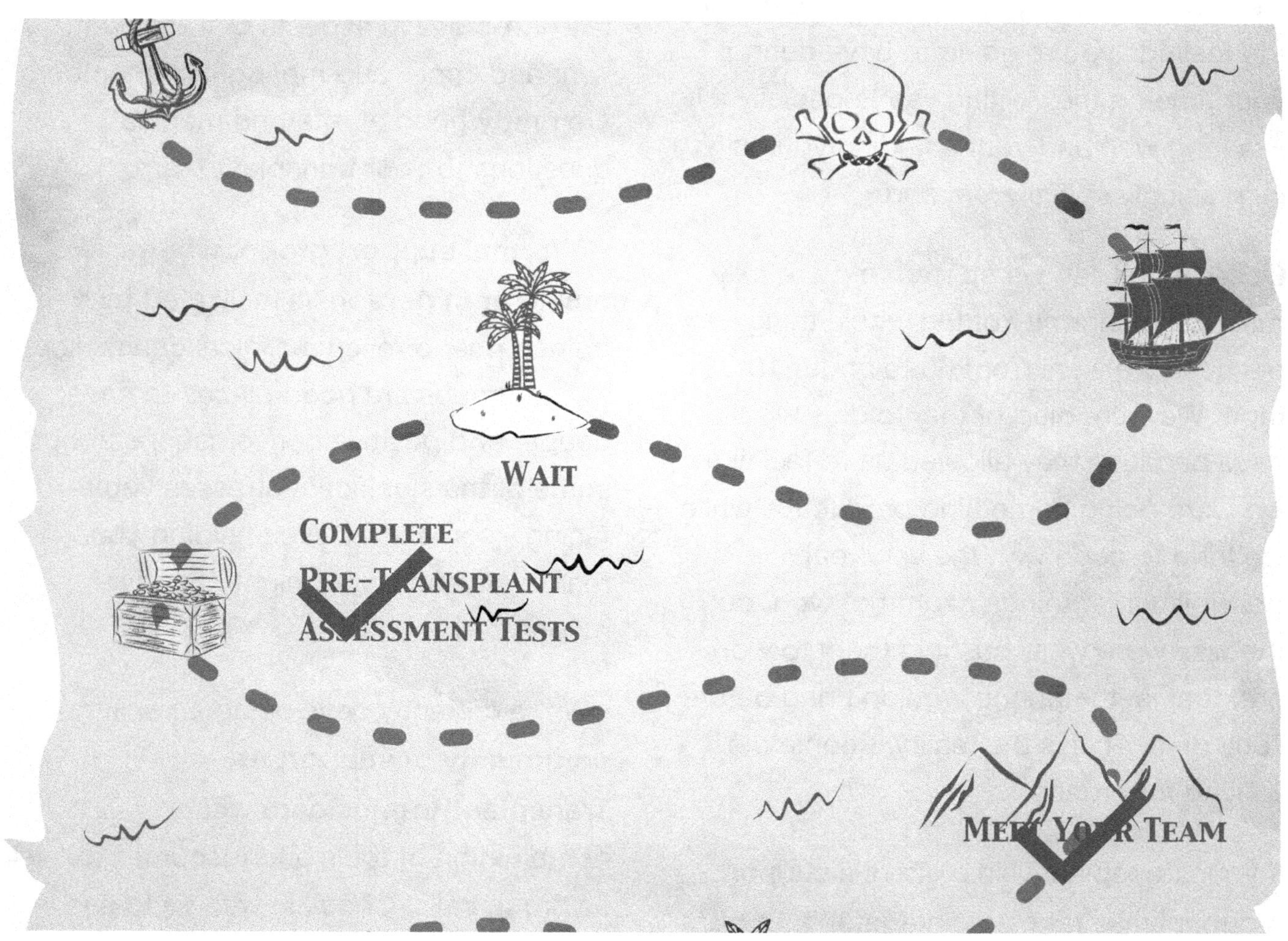

You will have some things to do in this stage, but by far the biggest issue for us was shifting from the crazy schedule of getting tests and procedures scheduled and completed to sitting around and worrying about the phone ringing.

Others have work to do in finding a suitable living donor. And then waiting for their surgery to be scheduled and actually happen.

You've done a significant amount of work to get to this point and the focus of your work changes.

It's important that you don't underestimate the feelings you're going to have during your time on the waiting list. Especially if it is a long wait and you're finding yourself increasingly socially isolated.

Once on the list, we started to more fully realize the enormity of the whole thing because we went from 60 to about 10 mph. We were glad of the 'to do's we did have because they allowed us to feel like we were doing something productive while we tried to cope with the very real possibility that things might not work out the way were were pushing them to work out: that is, the phone wouldn't ring before Tony died. This is the reality. People die waiting for organs.

If your Transplant Clinic offers a support group, please take advantage of it. **In our experience, getting connected with others who are patients and families was the best support resource. Find other support groups to join:**

• **Ask at your Transplant Clinic about in-person support group** and if it's live-streamed and/or supported online as a Facebook group (for example).

• **Informal online groups can be a great help**. They're a great place to ask about the non-medical aspects of transplant, vent and chat - and most group members are pretty good at referring medical questions to your transplant team.

• **A formal support group, whether online or in person**, is facilitated by a trained peer or even a clinical counsellor. These groups are good places to have deeper and positive conversations about some of the significant stresses you're facing - sometimes even helping you realize stressors you might not have recognized.

• We're currently developing an online **community of support at TransplantRogues.com** with a combination of tools and resources as well as group calls. Check in with us to see how to get involved.

Waiting List 'To Do's

There are a few key 'To Do's to focus on during your time on the waiting list:

• **Keep yourself healthy and fit**. Tony had a requirement for more protein to protect his muscle mass and we found a local physio rehab program for heart patients that we got him signed up for. Your transplant team will talk to you about your specific requirements. Get helpful tips from others in your support group(s).

• **Get your Go-bags packed**. We had go-bags packed and because we were also assuming we'd be gone for the full 3-6 months, we also had other items listed for packing once the phone rang (like Beth's work laptop, charger and files). We had 3 kinds of go-bags: Tony's hospital go-bag. Beth's longish-term go-bag and a go-bag for our accommodation with some food and kitchen items. This was waaayyyyy too much anxiety and overplanning. Pack a bag and throw in extras if/when you think about them. If you get caught short at the hospital, ask for help from the others in your group. If you're missing things from home, family and friends are waiting nervously in the wings to be given a task.

• **Make arrangements for being away** if this is your situation. At the minimum make sure that a few people have your house key so they can jump in and do what's needed. We agonized about finding a house-sitter and the stars aligned. Not because we agonized, but because we had our networks thinking about this early on in our journey.

Keep Your Binder Handy!

Be prepared, but don't panic about this. Plan what you can, but don't stress about the things you can't. We had no idea how we would find accommodation, but we did. The Transplant Team's Social Worker found us a place one block from the hospital. (Not to harp on a point but: connect, connect, connect with support groups. In the future it can be your turn to help out.)

Remember: You will land in an existing community among your transplant team and other recipient families. You can pick up supplies or have friends send or deliver things you may have forgotten. Your social worker knows all the secret accommodation places near the hospital. If not, then crowd-source answers through friends of friends. This is a time when having connections on social media can be invaluable.

Here are the things we made sure we had prepared so that we could travel with no notice if required:

1. We had a few spare keys cut and deployed them to friends and neighbours who would be in charge of the cats for a bit should we find ourselves caught short.

2. We had to drive to the ferry and then in to the hospital, so we made sure that the car's gas tank was always more than half-full because there's nothing open at night.

3. We made sure that Tony's oxygen tanks were always both as full as possible. Like the car, they were never allowed to go below 1/2 full.

4. We had the basics in Beth's purse. She kept a spare phone charger, her meds, spare pain meds for Tony, an envelope with 'go cash' and our travel documents* in her purse because she doesn't go anywhere without it. (We had a priority boarding card for the ferry should we have needed it.)

5. We had our binder!

#RoguesAreReady

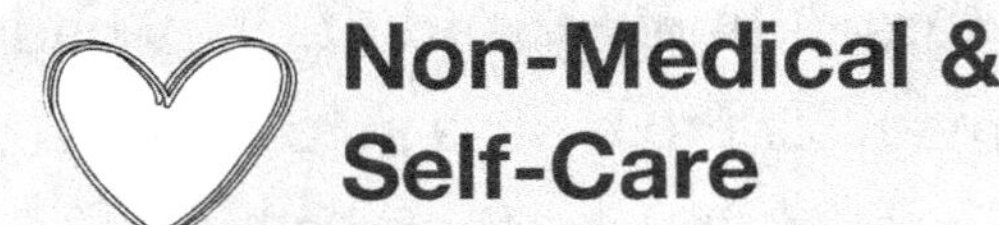

Non-Medical & Self-Care

The waiting list can be a challenge to your mental health, especially if you are finding yourself socially isolated.

One of the tools we use in our 'Empowered Patients & Families' workshop series is the 'Wellness Wheel'.

While your transplant team does everything they can to help you regain your physical health, it's important not to ignore the other aspects of your wellness.

Finding support can be difficult, and accessing support pre-transplant is even more difficult.

A friend of mine is launching a podcast series and started with a GREAT interview and resource for helping people keep their 'wellness wheels' from wobbling.

Check out her interview with counsellor Terry Folks and download the handouts here: https://karaforeman.com/podcast/wellnesswheel/

6

Recovery on the Transplant Unit

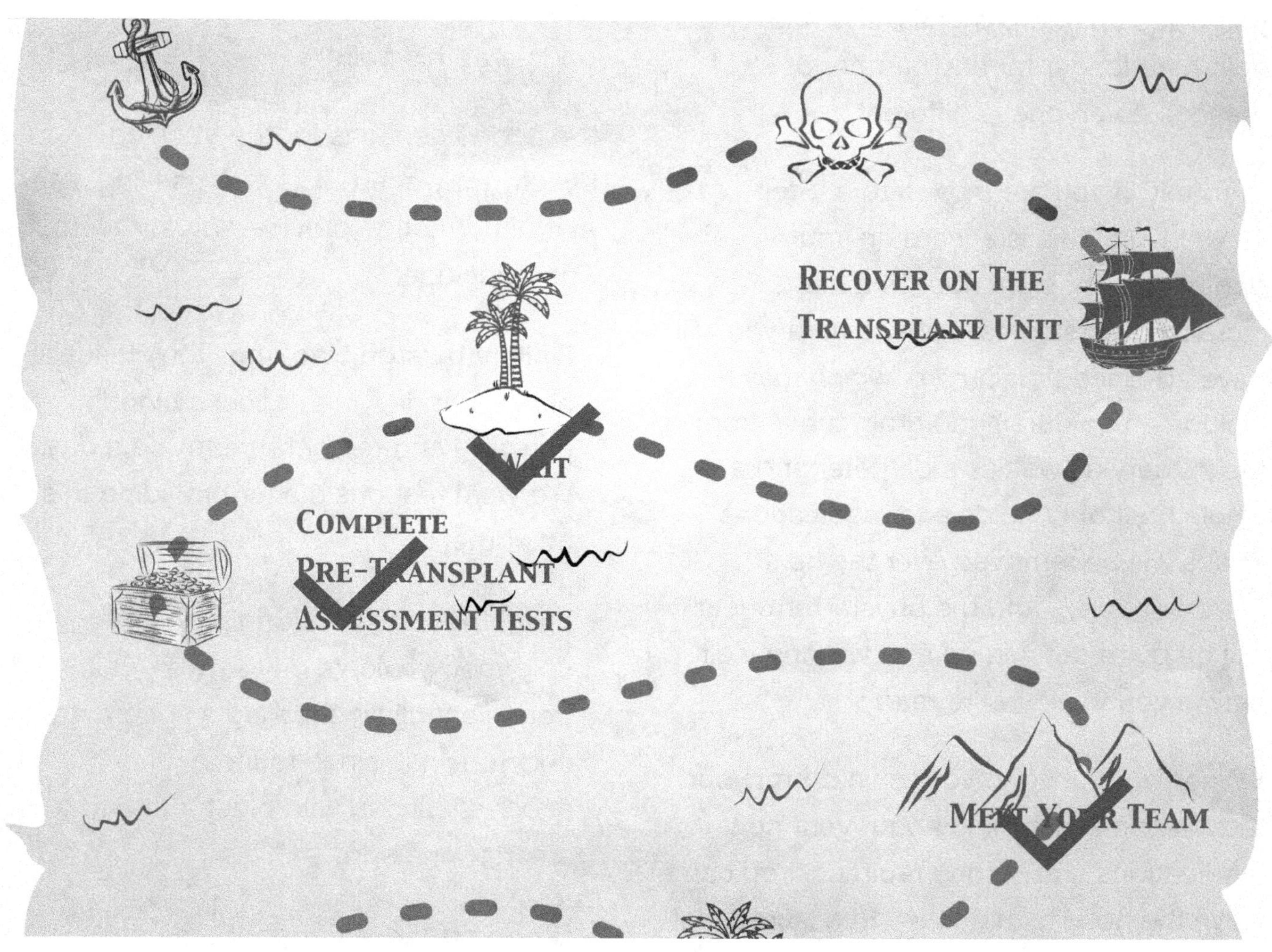

People's recover experiences post-transplant vary depending on countless factors. In general, after surgery you are moved to ICU and looked after there for a number of days during which time:

• You'll wake up with a breathing tube unless you're like Tony and yank it out while you're semi-conscious. This will be removed within a day or two. They'll let you know when you wake up.

• You'll be in ICU while you're on water, then clear fluids and then regular fluids (including Jello!) and then onto food. This lasts 2-5 days depending on how quickly you wake up and progress. You might be held here longer for any number of reasons. Everyone is different.

• From ICU you are moved to a 'Step-Down' Unit. This is a ward on your particular transplant floor that has increased nursing care. While here you will have advanced pain care (which may include an epidural) and drain tubes from the surgery as well as a catheter and a whole host of IV fluids and medications. These will be removed over the next number of days and the physio-terrorists will be by to get you up and walking well before you think you're ready.

• When you move to your own room, your task becomes learning about your new medications and testing regimes. You can't leave the hospital until they're assured that you and your caregiver are OK with medication dosages and timings and you can take your vital signs.

Rogues laugh at this last part because we're already doing a lot of this!

You just need to add a few more tracking sheets into your repertoire - and you'll get sheets from your Transplant team.

Patient and Caregiver Binder

Our patient binder underwent a radical update at this point!

We added sections for the tracking sheets Tony needed as well as filing extra information provided by our team. These include:

• **Daily vital sign tracking**. Tony takes his weight daily and checks blood pressure and temperature twice a day. We were responsible for providing this equipment.

• **Lung function tracking**. He does spirometry twice a day as well. Our transplant clinic supplied a spirometer and Tony has since found a super-small one with bluetooth and a smartphone app.

• **Blood sugar readings**. Fortunately, Tony left these behind when his prednisone dosage was cut in the year after transplant - but was doing these 3-4 times per day.

7

The First 3 Months

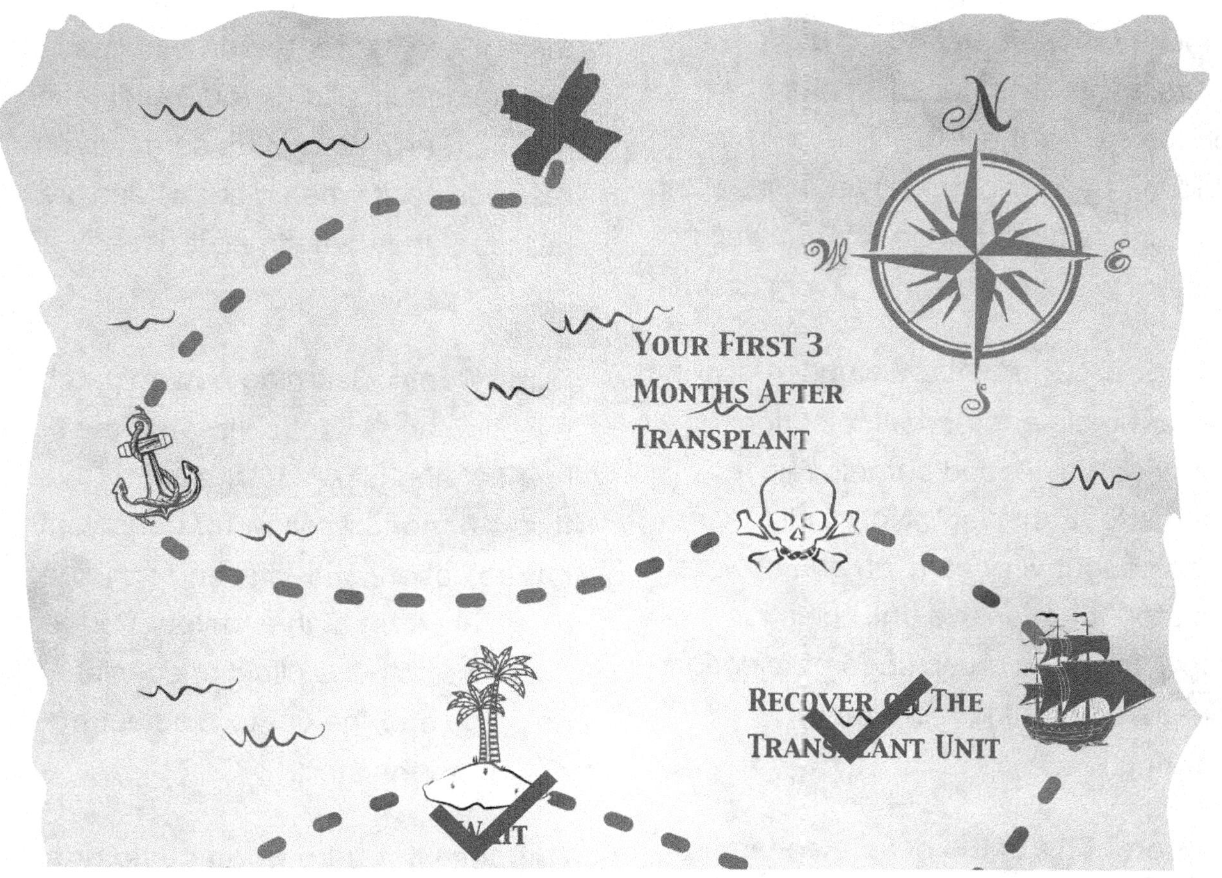

During the first 3 months, don't expect a catastrophe, but don't be surprised when you hit a bump. There are a lot of potential blips in the world of transplants and while serious and concerning, many are manageable. Catching things early is the key - so keeping up with your meds and vital sign tracking is the best habit you can develop.

Common 'Blips' that our gang encountered:

• Annoying Things Not Related to the Transplanted Organ - Tony's sternum didn't heal properly and 6 weeks after his transplant the team had to go back in and stabilize it with what look like bits of a Mechano set on the x-ray. This put him behind in physio (not good) and was a 2nd major surgery (also not good), but was not a problem with his transplant (very good).

• Rejection - One of the 2 elephants in the transplant recipient room is rejection. One of our gang developed chronic rejection 3 months after transplant. Not at all fun, but his was caught very early on and he was readmitted for intensive anti-rejection therapy. Tony had an episode of rejection that required nothing more than monitoring.

•Infection - This is the other elephant in the room. Common infections include CMV (cytomegalovirus) and an assortment of bacterial and viral infections. Like rejection, infections are potentially life-threatening and need to be caught early and treated with anti-virals and/or antibiotics. Again, this is where having good vital sign habits is very important.

• Steroid-Induced Hyperglycaemia (Diabetes) - One of the other common issues post-transplant is steroid-induced hyperglycaemia - a form of diabetes where your blood sugar rises throughout the day as a response to the prednisone you're taking. So you get to add blood-sugar testing and insulin to your medication regime. Fun? Wow! This sometimes resolves itself when medications are reduced and sometimes it doesn't. Fingers crossed!

Don't Panic - learning how to catch rejection and infection is what the first 3 months and clinics is all about. During the first 4-6 months following transplant your anti-rejection, anti-viral and antibiotic levels are kept high and your frequent checkins with the clinic are designed to help you and the doctors detect trouble right from the start.

Rogues who take good clinic notes and track their vitals are in good shape to handle the 'blips' when they occur!

#RoguesAreReady

8

The First Year: Rehab & Recovery

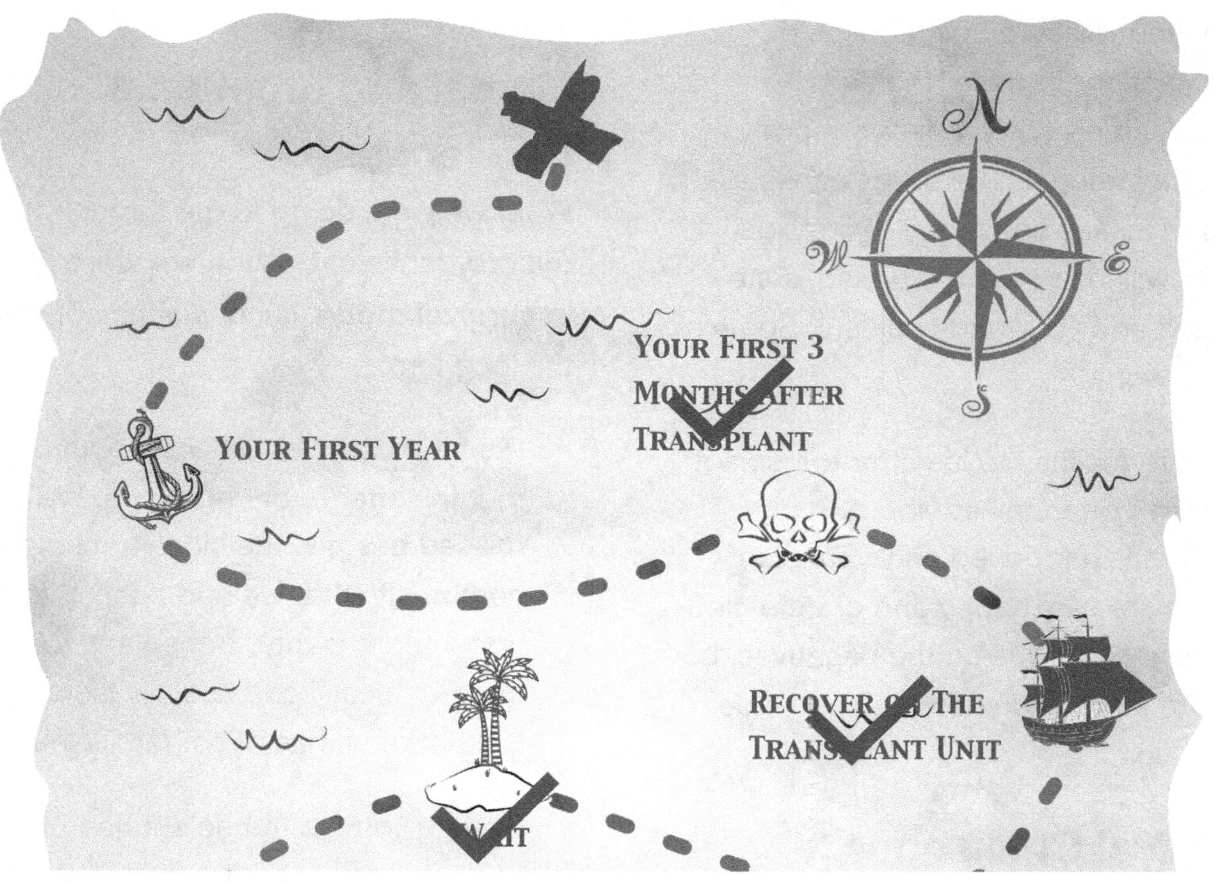

Transplant is NOT a cure. You will be living with transplant disease for the rest of your life. You will have good days and bad days. You will have clinic visits and more likely than not, hospital visits.

It might feel like there's a lot you can't do. But what you can do is focus on getting back on the road to living a more 'normal' life.

Some people are up and around fairly quickly and others aren't. It really does depend on a number of factors.

The first year is also the time when your body is doing a lot of work adjusting. Don't forget you will be on high doses of anti-rejection drugs for the first 3-6 months, so it's no wonder your body's having a struggle. The drugs cause all kinds of issues and many of the side effects will lessen as the dosages are reduced and your body adjusts. Some side effects won't.

There are realities to life after transplant that aren't often talked about. A big miracle has happened and transplant families are very happy and grateful and don't want to focus on the negatives, but they are there and you will experience them, too.

Physical Challenges

• Tony had pneumonia at 6 months post-transplant and again at 9 months that bought him another 2 weeks in hospital. **It's important to keep up with daily vital sign readings so you can pick up potential infection and rejection episodes and get in touch with your transplant clinic ASAP.**

• The post-transplant survival statistics have real-life impact for you now. So far we've had smooth sailing, but not everyone in Tony's cohort survived the first year. We feel the loss of our fellow warriors.

Mental and Emotional Challenges

What we were doing to get through things prior to transplant, **when we were literally in survival mode**, is not sustainable over the long term.

• We hit the proverbial wall about 3 months after returning home. We missed being in the close transplant community that we had been in for the first 4 months after transplant. We were geographically and socially isolated. Neither of us has direct family in BC.

• Getting Tony to transplant had used up our financial and emotional resources and once the immediate threat was over and we were alone, we ran headlong into depression. It's not uncommon after transplant and we now understand why. We had considerable difficulty finding effective mental health supports. This is an area that needs some serious attention if we are to help transplant patients and families move more quickly towards 'living life again'.

- Additionally, since Tony was getting well instead of dying, all of his other medical issues were now being addressed. We had referrals to Complex Pain, Rheumatology, Ophthalmology, Dermatology, Occupational Therapy, Physiotherapy and Psychology (for insomnia, not depression even though we kept mentioning it). We still lived a minimum 30 minute drive out of the nearest town. Beth couldn't continue to be a full-time caregiver and drive Tony to these appointments. And Tony was unable to do the amount of driving required.

- We made the decision to move to a major centre so Beth could find work and Tony could get himself to appointments. It meant we could no longer own our own home and had to begin to cope with having to restart not just financially, but socially.

- By Tony's first 'Lungaversary' we had just listed our house for sale. Our road to 'living life again' was still long. We had significant challenges in just about every area of transplant. We sincerely hope the challenges other Rogues face - and the gaps they fall through - are fewer.

Upshot: You may need to make - and cope with - some major life changes after transplant.

We saw early in our journey the other patients and family caregivers who were struggling with the intense learning curve for the medical aspects of the transplant journey. Tony, too, had questions that I was able to answer, and from that we created the information on Transplant Rogues.

What we didn't see coming was the enormous damage to our own mental (and then financial) health as a result of the decade of Tony's declining physical health and subsequent life-saving transplant. We were like the frogs in the boiling water story - we were in survival mode and coped the best we could until we couldn't cope any longer.

We asked for, and were ignored or denied help from the system often enough prior to transplant that we had stopped asking and assumed it was unavailable.

Part of that was a result of living outside a major centre. Access to support services is just not as available in smaller centres as it is in larger cities. For example, our transplant clinic runs a support group - but it's only accessible for people living in Vancouver. The **patients** in Vancouver set up a Facebook group to communicate among themselves and they invite new transplant recipients to join - but it's not formally run by the transplant clinic.

At the end of our first year post-transplant we were still very much 'up in the air'.

Things were to get somewhat more challenging for our second year - but I'll end this chapter with a 'spoiler alert'.

It gets better!

9

The Second Year & Beyond

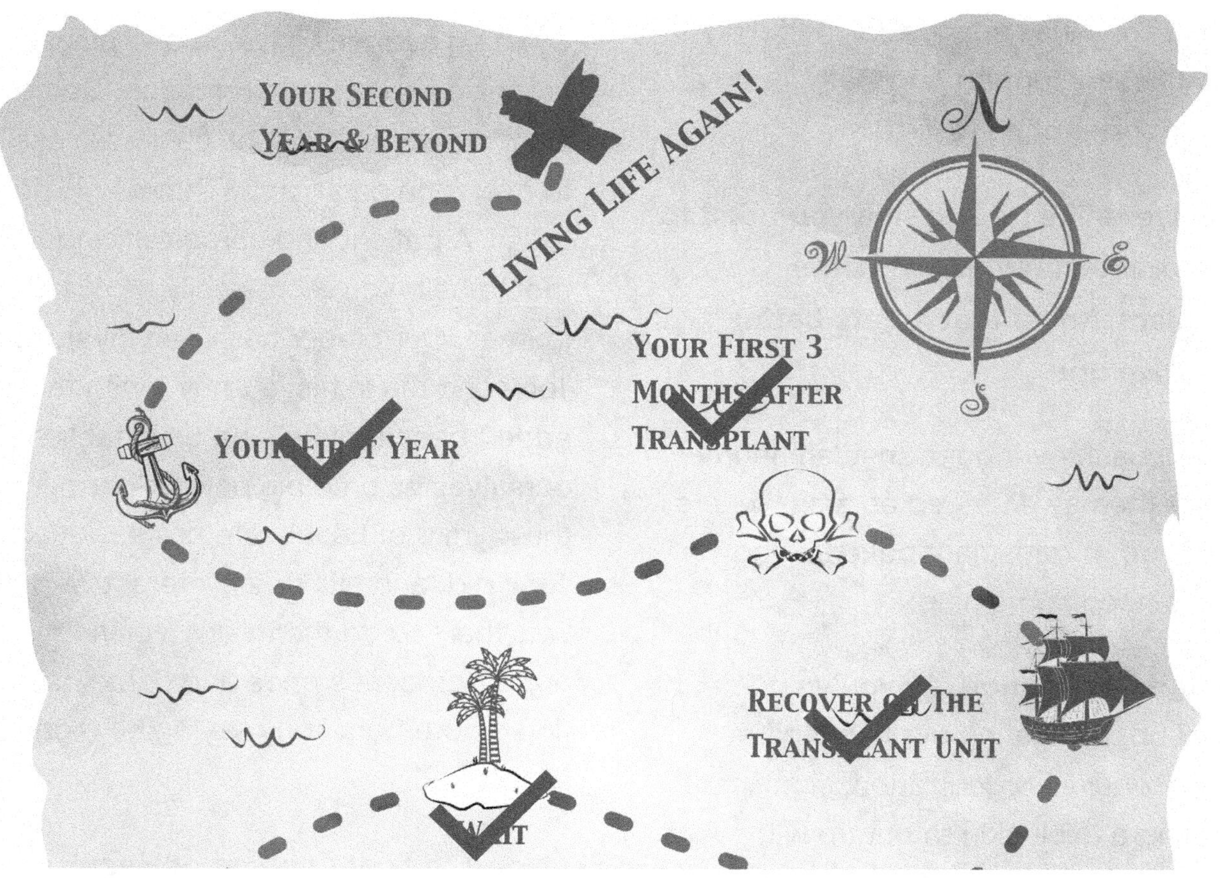

Transplant patients and families often face difficult issues that we need help to process before we can effectively move on to living life again.

By the end of our second year we had moved, were coming to terms with our new living situation and were getting settled in to a more sustainable lifestyle.

As we found ourselves in a larger centre, we were able to connect with the medical follow-up care Tony needed, and the logistics of getting to and from all his appointments was significantly easier.

Further, Tony was successful in finding mental health support and Beth found a few support groups to join.

If you were like us and find you need to make drastic life changes after transplant, know that it gets better. Don't give up!

Looking back over our transplant journey, 3 major themes emerged as areas where we and other transplant patients and families need some help:

• **System Navigation**. As you've no doubt picked up, navigating our healthcare system requires organization, significant time, and a thick skin to put up with what can often become a frustrating and demoralizing process. There's a steep learning curve that we need to navigate - without training, without pay and at the most stressful point of our lives. System navigation is an ongoing responsibility that can leave Rogues feeling isolated, distressed and even traumatized. **Dealing with the healthcare system over the**

long term is made easier when you can pick up some basic skills and you have others who have lived through it to speak with.

• **Patient and Caregiver Binder** - Creating a binder gave us one place to organize and store information. Some day, all of our records will be easily accessible to everyone on an app. That day is not today. A patient and caregiver binder is a tool to help you more easily navigate your journey. Our binder has been invaluable to Tony and me in his journey - with the added benefit of helping us establish ourselves as credible patient-partners with the myriad of healthcare professionals Tony did, and still does, interact with. It was there to do the talking when I went out for groceries once and came back to find a note from Tony saying he'd called 911.

• **Non-Medical Aspects of Health & Self-Care** - The healthcare system doesn't see patients - let alone their distressed family caregivers - as whole people. You will run across wonderful people working within the system, some of whom will bend rules to help - but the system itself is always there. The system sees mental health as completely separate from physical health, and in the hierarchy of medical specialties, psychology is at the bottom. In British Columbia we have completely separate government ministries for health and mental health. And with the exception of psychiatry and some short-term intervention programs, mental health supports are not covered by our Medical Services Plan - meaning mental health supports are seen as unnecessary for health. As a result, when you are on a long-term healthcare journey you are unlikely to have your mental health needs considered, let alone acknowledged and supported.

For patients and families, mental health aspect is an issue at every stop along the transplant journey. It falls to us to do what we can for ourselves.

As transplant patients and families, we absolutely need to come together as a community regardless of organ of transplant.

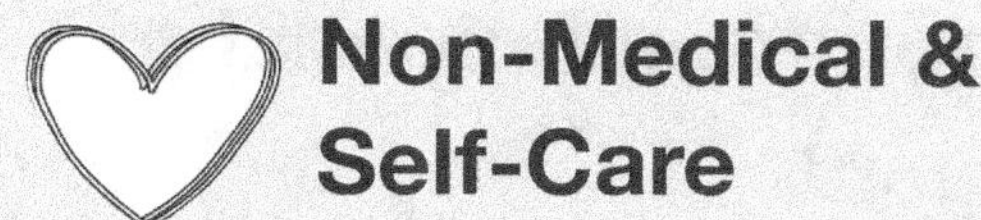

Non-Medical & Self-Care

We are working on in-person workshops and online coaching to help Rogues:

• Learn how to more easily navigate our healthcare system,

• Create and use their patient and caregiver binders, and

• Figure out how to find and access their local resources.

We can't magically create a better, less distressing healthcare and social support system, but we can sure as hell work together - regardless of organ of transplant - to share resources, stories and support.

You know where to find us - and to refer other Rogues:

TransplantRogues.com

The Enormous Potential of Transplant

Transplant is a medical miracle. It's developed medically in a relatively short period of time.

Transplant has developed in leaps and bounds - not just in our lifetimes, but in Tony and Beth's ADULT lifetimes.

Long-term patients and families bring their whole selves into healthcare. They bring their hopes. They bring their pain.

Transplant patients are more than lungs and livers and kidneys. Transplant care must include more than just lungs and livers and kidneys. It has to start acknowledging the distress in which patients and families arrive in their care - and the further distress and trauma that is caused by the process.

As one long-term lung transplant recipient said to me: PTSD. We all have it, but nobody wants to fucking talk about it.

Transplant doesn't just impact the patient. It has significant impacts on the designated family caregiver and the greater family unit. If transplant is to avoid creating more patients for the healthcare -

and subsequently the social welfare - system, it needs to make the shift from the bureaucracy-centred model we have now to being truly patient and family directed.

Transplant clinics have enormous potential to be leaders in the healthcare system's shift towards patient-centred, mental health-informed, careful and kind care. Once we make this shift, transplant can be truly transformative.

Until that day, Rogues, it's critical that we:

- Seek each other out,

- Talk about the hard things, and

- Support each other.

Find us at: TransplantRogues.com

10

Patient & Family Caregiver Handouts

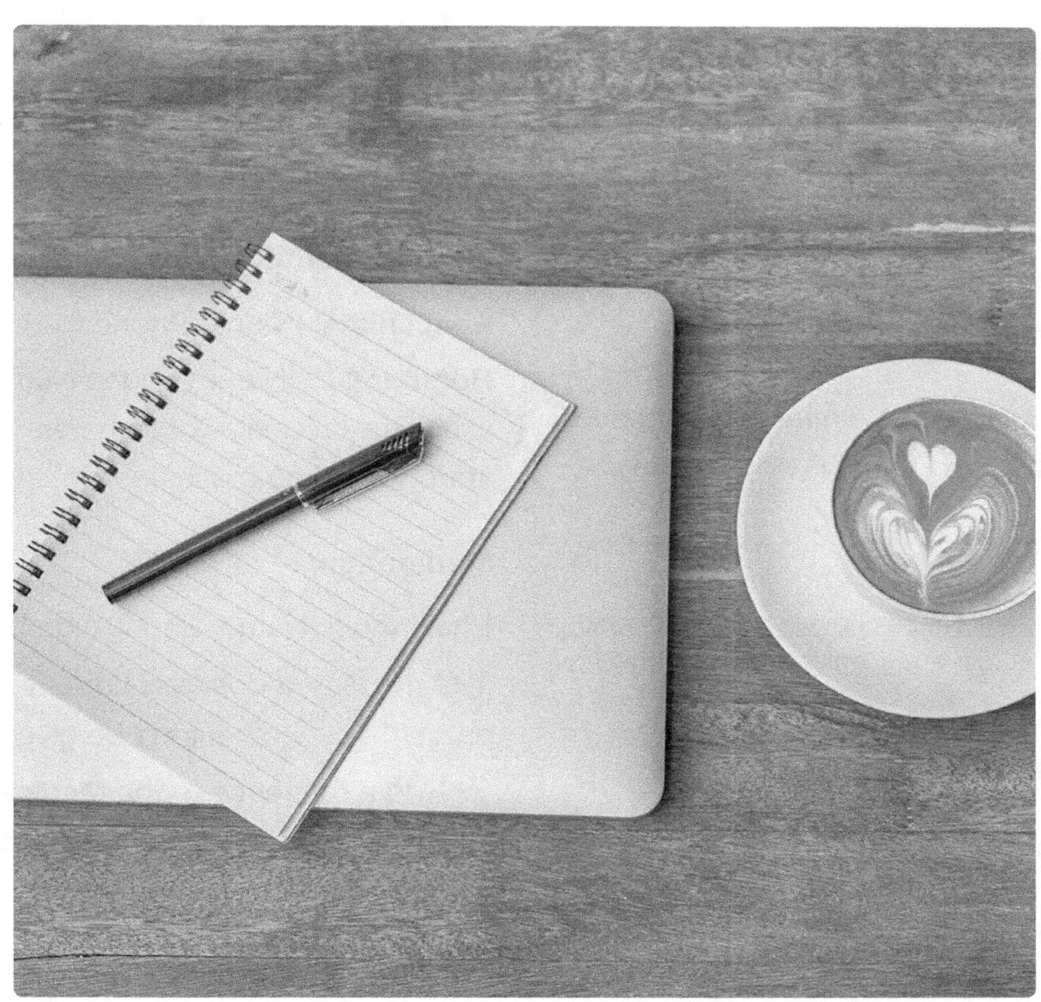

Patient One-Page Summary

Tony's summary is the first page of his binder. We put it into a plastic sheet protector.

This is invaluable for emergencies and helpful at new doctors' appointments as it lists his name, health number, current diagnoses, medications and emergency contact information.

We hustled ours up in a Word document so we can update it easily and print out a fresh copy when needed.

We also keep all of our information sheets in a DropBox that we can each access on our phones if necessary.

Some day, this will be digital and attached to your CareCard. Today is not that day.

Download a Word document that you can fill in directly here:
http://transplantrogues.com/wp-content/uploads/2016/09/Medical-and-Contact-Information-Sheet.docx

My Name
Cell
Health #
D.O.B.

Medical Conditions: [Include special instructions - like 'requires oxygen' and any allergies]

[Listed, Being Assessed, Recipient] for [kind of] transplant at [Name of] Hospital

Contact: [Coordinator's name]
Tel: [Contact Number(s)]
After Hours: [Coordinator Pager Number once listed]

Medical Contacts:

Specialists: [Name, Phone Numbers]
Regular GP: [Name, Phone Numbers - clinic, on-call cell, Doctor's cell. They will start giving you these.]

Medications:

Pharmacy: [Name, Phone Number]
[List meds and dosages here - include any drugs that you shouldn't be given]

• Add a reference to the Medication Summary Sheet if/when this list gets too long to fit here.

Emergency contacts: [Name, Phone Number]

Members: My Transplant Team

Role	Name	Phone	Email	Notes
Local Team				
General Practitioner				
Specialist				
Pharmacist				
Transplant Team				
Transplant Physicians				
Transplant Nurses				
Transplant Coordinator				
Transplant Surgeon				
Psychologist				
Dietician				
Social Worker				
Other Health Contacts				

Medication List

We used a variety of formats for our Medication List and eventually settled on this format for 2 reasons:

1. Tony's medications became too complex for a simple list with the medication name and dosage. Timing of medications became an issue because some meds can't be taken together.
2. This format is the one used by our hospital, and we had medication reconciliation issues more often than not when Tony was hospitalized. Using this format helps minimize errors.

Customize the columns for your own medication schedule.

You can find an Excel spreadsheet that you can customise at: http://transplantrogues.com/wp-content/uploads/2016/08/Transplant-Rogues-Medication-Summary.xlsx

Medication	Dose	Indication	8 am	Noon	5 pm	8 pm
Mycophenolate	1500 mg twice daily	Anti-rejection	X			X
Calcium citrate	600 mg twice daily	Required supplement		X	X	

Clinic Notes

Date	Notes	Status
	Issue	
	Resolution	
	Issue	
	Resolution	
	Issue	
	Resolution	
	Issue	
	Resolution	
	Issue	
	Resolution	
	Issue	
	Resolution	
	Issue	
	Resolution	
	Issue	
	Resolution	

5 Questions to ask your health-care professionals ~ From *How Doctors Think* (Jerome Groopman)

♦ What else could it be? ♦ Is there anything that doesn't fit? ♦ Is it possible I have more than one problem?

♦ Tell the doctor what you are most worried about. ♦ Retell the story from the beginning (if the issue isn't being resolved)